Dash Diet Cookbook For Beginners 2024

Achieve Your Health Goals with Flavorful DASH Diet Meals at Your Fingertips

McDonnell B. Young

Table of Contents

Introduction   5

   What is the DASH Diet?   8

   Benefits of the DASH Diet   11

   How to Use This Cookbook   14

Chapter: 1 Breakfast Recipes   17

   Oatmeal with Fresh Berries and Nuts   17

   Greek Yogurt Parfait with Muesli and Honey   19

   Spinach and Feta Egg Muffins   21

   Banana Pancakes with Maple Yogurt   23

   Avocado Toast with Poached Eggs   25

   Smoothie Bowl with Chia Seeds and Kiwi   27

   Whole Wheat Blueberry Waffles   29

   Cottage Cheese with Pineapple and Chia   31

   Breakfast Quinoa with Apples and Cinnamon   33

   Veggie Omelette with Mushrooms and Tomatoes   35

Chapter: 2 Lunch Recipes   37

   Quinoa Salad with Chickpeas and Feta   37

   Grilled Vegetable and Hummus Wraps   40

   Turkey and Avocado Club Sandwich   42

   Mixed Bean Soup with Barley   44

   Spinach and Strawberry Salad with Walnuts   47

   Tuna Salad Stuffed Tomatoes   49

Chicken Caesar Salad with Whole Grain Croutons 51

Mediterranean Veggie Pita Sandwich 54

Butternut Squash and Apple Soup 56

Roasted Beet and Citrus Salad 58

Chapter: 3 Dinner Recipes 60

Baked Salmon with Dill and Lemon 60

Grilled Chicken with Quinoa and Broccoli 62

Vegetable Stir-Fry with Tofu and Brown Rice 64

Beef Stew with Root Vegetables 67

Pasta Primavera with a Light Tomato Sauce 69

Pork Tenderloin with Roasted Sweet Potatoes 72

Seafood Paella with Brown Rice 75

Eggplant Parmesan Light 78

Turkey Chili with Beans 80

Lentil and Spinach Curry 82

Chapter: 4 Snacks and Sides 85

Healthy Snack Options 85

Sides to Complement Your Meals 90

Chapter: 5 Desserts 94

Sweet Treats That Fit the DASH Diet 94

Chapter: 6 Drinks and Beverages 98

Refreshing Drinks for Hydration and Health 98

Conclusion 102

Introduction

Jane Thompson glanced at the kitchen clock, sighing as her physician's words echoed in her head, "You need to control your hypertension, Jane. I suggest looking into the DASH diet." Hypertension was her unwanted companion, tagging along through her stressful days and sleepless nights. Her journey to better health seemed daunting until she discovered the "DASH Diet Cookbook For Beginners 2024" at her local bookstore.

The vibrant cover, featuring an array of colorful, heart-healthy foods, beckoned. Hesitant but hopeful, Jane skimmed the table of contents, impressed by the thorough breakdown from breakfast to dinner, including snacks and desserts all catered to the DASH diet. It wasn't just recipes; the book promised a guide on how to transform her eating habits. Taking a deep breath, she made the purchase that would pivot her life's direction.

Back home, Jane explored the first chapter, which detailed what the DASH diet was and its benefits—specifically how it could reduce blood pressure and improve heart health. It wasn't preachy; it felt like a friend walking her through the science in simple terms. The pages on essential ingredients and kitchen tools were equally enlightening, making her feel equipped, not overwhelmed.

She started with breakfast, opting for the Spinach and Feta Egg Muffins. The recipe was straightforward, and to her delight, delicious. Energized by her success, she planned her week around the book's meal plans, each day experimenting with different recipes like the Quinoa Salad with Chickpeas for lunch and Baked Salmon with Dill for dinner. The book even offered heart-healthy snack ideas that were perfect for her mid-afternoon cravings.

Each recipe Jane tried was a revelation, bursting with flavor and yet, simple to prepare. Her apprehension about bland dietary food dissolved with each spice-infused, herb-sprinkled dish. The grocery shopping tips and meal prep strategies outlined in the book streamlined her cooking process, making it less time-consuming and more enjoyable.

Weeks turned into months, and Jane found herself more energetic, her blood pressure readings steadily improving. The unexpected gem was the chapter on dining out, which equipped her with the knowledge to make smart, DASH-friendly choices in restaurants without feeling deprived.

One evening, as she sipped a homemade herbal tea detailed in the beverage section, Jane reflected on her journey. The "DASH Diet Cookbook For Beginners 2024" had been more than just a collection of recipes; it was a mentor. It had gently steered her through a transformation that was not only about losing weight or lowering blood pressure but about gaining vitality and joy.

As her friends began to notice her renewed vigor and glowing health, Jane recommended the cookbook with a passionate zeal. "It's not just about following a diet," she would say, "It's about learning to enjoy life with every nutritious meal you make."

For anyone standing at the crossroads of health concerns and dietary change, Jane's story is a testament to how the right guide can open a path to wellness and empowerment. The "DASH Diet Cookbook For Beginners 2024" is not just a purchase; it's an investment in a healthier, happier future.

What is the DASH Diet?

The DASH Diet, which stands for Dietary Approaches to Stop Hypertension, is a lifelong approach to healthy eating designed to help treat or prevent high blood pressure (hypertension). Developed in the early 1990s through research sponsored by the U.S. National Institutes of Health, this diet emphasizes the consumption of fruits, vegetables, whole grains, and lean proteins, while reducing the intake of sodium, red meat, sweets, and sugary beverages. It is not only backed by scientific research but also highly recommended by health professionals for its effectiveness in lowering blood pressure and improving overall health.

Unlike many fad diets that focus on rapid weight loss, the DASH diet is recognized for its balanced and sustainable approach, making it particularly beneficial for beginners. It promotes gradual changes in eating habits, encouraging individuals to reduce portion sizes, consume a variety of nutrient-rich foods, and limit foods high in saturated fat and sugar. This comprehensive approach not only helps in managing blood pressure but also supports a healthy weight and reduces the risk of diabetes, cancer, and other chronic diseases.

In the "DASH Diet Cookbook For Beginners 2024," the principles of the DASH diet are tailored for those who are new to this eating plan. The cookbook provides a practical and easy-to-follow framework that introduces the diet's core components through delicious, simple recipes. Each recipe is designed to meet specific nutritional guidelines, ensuring that users can enjoy a wide range of flavors while sticking to the health objectives of the DASH diet.

The inclusion of detailed nutritional information with each recipe is a key feature of the cookbook, helping beginners understand the nutritional impact of each meal. This not only aids in following the diet but also educates the reader on making healthier food choices. The cookbook also offers alternatives and modifications for common recipes, accommodating various tastes and dietary restrictions while maintaining nutritional integrity.

One of the standout features of the DASH diet is its flexibility in dietary choices, which is well captured in the cookbook. Whether a person is a vegetarian, has a gluten intolerance, or prefers organic foods, the cookbook provides options that can be tailored to fit these needs. This adaptability makes it easier for individuals to adopt and maintain the diet as part of a permanent lifestyle change rather than a temporary dietary experiment.

For beginners, starting a new diet can be challenging, especially when it comes to meal planning and preparation. The "DASH Diet Cookbook For Beginners 2024" addresses this challenge by including sample meal plans and shopping lists. These resources simplify the process of integrating the DASH diet into daily life, making it less daunting for newcomers. The meal plans are designed to gradually introduce the diet's principles, easing the transition and helping individuals make lasting dietary changes.

Finally, the cookbook emphasizes the importance of a supportive eating environment. It encourages cooking at home and sharing meals with family and friends, which not only enhances the enjoyment of food but also reinforces the adoption of healthier eating habits. Through its comprehensive and thoughtful approach, the "DASH Diet Cookbook For Beginners 2024" serves as an invaluable guide for anyone looking to improve their health through dietary changes, providing the tools and knowledge necessary to embark on a journey toward better health with confidence.

Benefits of the DASH Diet

The DASH diet, which stands for Dietary Approaches to Stop Hypertension, is a long-celebrated eating plan endorsed by numerous health experts for its effectiveness in lowering blood pressure and promoting overall cardiovascular health. Rooted in a balance of nutrient-rich foods, the diet emphasizes fruits, vegetables, whole grains, lean proteins, and low-fat dairy, while reducing the intake of fats, red meats, and sweets. This approach not only aids in managing blood pressure but also supports a healthy weight and strengthens the immune system by providing a diverse range of essential vitamins and minerals.

In the "DASH Diet Cookbook For Beginners 2024," the principles of this nutritious diet are made accessible to those who might be new to health-conscious cooking. The cookbook presents a practical pathway for integrating the DASH diet into daily life without the need for drastic lifestyle changes. It offers a variety of recipes that include all the food groups recommended in the diet, ensuring that meals are balanced and rich in flavor. This diversity helps to stave off dietary boredom and encourages adherence to the eating plan, enhancing its effectiveness.

The book also delves into the benefits of the DASH diet in regulating cholesterol levels. By limiting the intake of unhealthy fats and focusing on fiber-rich foods, the diet naturally combats high levels of LDL (bad) cholesterol. Lower cholesterol is directly linked to reduced risks of heart disease and stroke, illustrating the DASH diet's role in long-term heart health. This aspect is particularly beneficial for those with a family history of heart-related issues, providing a proactive approach to disease prevention through diet.

Another significant advantage of the DASH diet explored in the cookbook is its impact on insulin sensitivity. The high fiber content in whole grains and legumes slows the absorption of sugar, helping to regulate blood sugar levels. This is crucial for the prevention and management of diabetes, a common concern that often accompanies hypertension. By demonstrating how to prepare meals that support blood sugar control, the cookbook serves as a valuable resource for those looking to manage or prevent diabetes.

Weight management is another area where the DASH diet proves advantageous. The cookbook highlights how the diet's emphasis on vegetables and fruits, which are low in calories but high in fiber, helps individuals feel fuller longer. This natural appetite control facilitates a lower calorie intake and can lead to sustainable weight loss. The recipes provided ensure that users do not feel deprived, making it easier to maintain a healthy weight without resorting to drastic or unhealthy measures.

The cookbook also addresses the reduction of sodium intake, which is a cornerstone of the DASH diet. Excessive sodium is a known contributor to hypertension, and the diet's focus on fresh, unprocessed foods naturally diminishes sodium consumption. Through creative seasoning alternatives and the use of herbs and spices, the recipes ensure that meals are delicious and full of flavor without relying on salt. This not only benefits blood pressure levels but also enhances the overall palate, allowing the natural tastes of food to shine through.

Finally, "DASH Diet Cookbook For Beginners 2024" supports mental health by promoting a diet rich in nutrients associated with brain health, such as omega-3 fatty acids from fish and antioxidants from berries and nuts. The stress of managing hypertension and other health issues can be overwhelming, but following a diet that also supports mental well-being can provide a significant psychological boost. This holistic approach to health, which includes both physical and mental benefits, is what makes the DASH diet and the cookbook an essential tool for those beginning their journey towards a healthier life.

How to Use This Cookbook

The "DASH Diet Cookbook For Beginners 2024" is crafted to guide you through a transformative journey toward healthier eating habits, specifically designed to help manage and prevent hypertension. It's structured to gradually introduce the fundamentals of the Dietary Approaches to Stop Hypertension, or DASH, diet, providing not just the 'what' but the 'why' behind the choice of ingredients and methods. Each recipe is meticulously developed to ensure it meets the nutritional guidelines without sacrificing flavor, making the transition to healthier eating seamless and enjoyable.

For those unfamiliar with kitchen basics or the specific demands of a health-focused diet, the cookbook includes detailed descriptions of kitchen tools and essential ingredients that form the backbone of the DASH diet. This ensures that before you begin any recipe, you're fully prepared with the right equipment and pantry staples. This preparation is crucial for making cooking less daunting and more efficient, which is particularly helpful for beginners.

The recipes themselves are designed with flexibility in mind, catering to varying skill levels and time constraints. They range from quick, simple dishes to more elaborate meals, each marked with prep and cooking times. This allows you to choose recipes that fit into your schedule, whether you're looking for a quick breakfast before work or a more involved dinner when you have more time to indulge in the cooking process.

Portion control is a significant aspect of the DASH diet, and the cookbook emphasizes this through clear, easy-to-follow serving suggestions. Understanding portion sizes is vital for managing blood pressure and overall health, and the cookbook helps you visualize and measure portions without the need for complicated calculations or specialist equipment.

Meal planning is another key feature addressed in the cookbook. By providing a week's worth of meal plans that utilize a variety of recipes from the book, it demonstrates how to effectively prepare meals without last-minute stress. This not only saves time but also ensures that you stick to the diet by having healthy options at hand. The meal plans are designed to be adaptable, allowing you to swap meals depending on your preference, which keeps the diet flexible and realistic for everyday life.

Understanding that everyone's palate and dietary needs can differ, the cookbook encourages modifications to recipes. It offers suggestions on how to substitute ingredients to cater to allergies, personal taste, or even seasonal availability. This not only helps in personalizing the diet to your liking but also teaches the principles of healthy substitutions that can be applied beyond the recipes provided.

Finally, the cookbook emphasizes the importance of reflection and adjustment. It encourages you to monitor how the changes in diet affect your health and well-being, suggesting regular check-ins with yourself and potentially your healthcare provider. This reflection can help you adapt the diet to better meet your health goals and preferences, making the DASH diet a sustainable and beneficial part of your lifestyle rather than just a temporary change.

Chapter: 1 Breakfast Recipes

Oatmeal with Fresh Berries and Nuts

Ingredients:

- 1 cup rolled oats
- 2 cups water or low-fat milk for creamier texture
- 1/2 cup mixed berries (blueberries, strawberries, and raspberries)
- 1/4 cup chopped nuts (almonds, walnuts, or pecans)
- 1 tablespoon honey or maple syrup (optional)
- 1/2 teaspoon cinnamon

Instructions:

1. In a medium saucepan, bring the water or milk to a boil.
2. Add the rolled oats and cinnamon, reducing heat to a simmer. Stir occasionally, cooking for about 5 minutes until the oats are soft and have absorbed most of the liquid.
3. Remove the cooked oats from the heat and let them sit for two minutes to thicken further.
4. Serve the oatmeal in bowls topped with fresh berries, nuts, and a drizzle of honey or maple syrup if desired.

Nutritional Information:

Each serving of this oatmeal provides a nutrient-rich meal with approximately 300 calories, 8 grams of fiber, and 10 grams of protein. The inclusion of nuts adds healthy fats that are good for heart health, while the berries provide essential vitamins and antioxidants.

Serving Size:

This recipe serves two. It's perfect for a filling single serving or can be shared for a lighter meal, making it versatile depending on your dietary needs.

Cooking Time:

The total cooking time for this recipe is about 10 minutes, which includes the time to bring the liquid to a boil and the time needed for the oats to cook and thicken. This makes it an ideal quick and easy meal for busy mornings.

Greek Yogurt Parfait with Muesli and Honey

For the Greek Yogurt Parfait with Muesli and Honey, you'll need the following ingredients:

- 1 cup low-fat Greek yogurt
- 1/2 cup muesli
- 1 tablespoon honey
- 1/2 cup mixed berries (such as blueberries, strawberries, and raspberries)
- A sprinkle of cinnamon (optional for added flavor)

Instructions are straightforward to ensure a quick and easy preparation process:

1. In a serving glass or bowl, layer half of the Greek yogurt at the bottom.
2. Add a layer of half the muesli over the yogurt.
3. Drizzle half of the honey over the muesli.
4. Add half of the mixed berries as the next layer.
5. Repeat the layering process with the remaining yogurt, muesli, honey, and berries.

6. Top with a sprinkle of cinnamon if desired for extra flavor.

7. Serve immediately or refrigerate overnight for an enhanced melding of flavors.

The nutritional information for this recipe is particularly beneficial for those monitoring their intake for health reasons:

- Calories: 320
- Total Fat: 2g
- Saturated Fat: 1g
- Cholesterol: 10mg
- Sodium: 50mg
- Carbohydrates: 53g
- Fiber: 4g
- Sugars: 30g (includes 12g added sugars)
- Protein: 20g

Each **serving size** consists of one full glass or bowl of the parfait, perfectly portioned to satisfy as a complete breakfast meal.

The **cooking time** is minimal, with the total preparation time being approximately 5 minutes. This makes the Greek Yogurt Parfait with Muesli and Honey an excellent choice for a nutritious, quick, and easy breakfast option

Spinach and Feta Egg Muffins

Ingredients:

- 6 large eggs
- 1 cup fresh spinach, chopped
- 1/2 cup feta cheese, crumbled
- 1/4 cup onions, finely diced
- 1/4 cup skim milk
- Salt and pepper to taste (minimal salt for DASH compliance)
- Cooking spray or a dab of olive oil for the muffin tin

Instructions:

1. Preheat your oven to 375 degrees Fahrenheit (190 degrees Celsius).
2. Lightly grease a 6-cup muffin tin with cooking spray or olive oil.
3. In a mixing bowl, whisk the eggs and milk together until well combined.
4. Stir in the chopped spinach, diced onions, and crumbled feta cheese.
5. Season with a pinch of salt and pepper.
6. Pour the egg mixture evenly into the prepared muffin tin.
7. Bake in the preheated oven for 20-25 minutes, or until the egg muffins are firm to the touch and cooked through.

Cooking Time:

- Total preparation and cooking time is approximately 30-35 minutes.

Serving Size:

- This recipe makes 6 muffins, with a recommended serving size of 2 muffins per person.

Nutritional Information per Serving:

- Calories: Approximately 150
- Total Fat: 10g
- Saturated Fat: 4g
- Cholesterol: 215mg
- Sodium: 220mg
- Total Carbohydrates: 3g
- Dietary Fiber: 0.5g
- Sugars: 2g
- Protein: 12g

Banana Pancakes with Maple Yogurt

Ingredients:

- 1 cup whole wheat flour
- 1 tablespoon sugar (optional)
- 2 teaspoons baking powder
- 1/2 teaspoon salt
- 1 egg, beaten
- 1 cup non-fat milk
- 2 ripe bananas, mashed
- 1/2 teaspoon vanilla extract
- Non-stick cooking spray or a small amount of olive oil for cooking
- 1/2 cup Greek yogurt
- 2 tablespoons pure maple syrup

Instructions:

1. In a large bowl, combine the flour, sugar (if using), baking powder, and salt.
2. In another bowl, whisk together the beaten egg, milk, mashed bananas, and vanilla extract.
3. Pour the wet ingredients into the dry ingredients, stirring until the mixture is just combined. Be careful not to overmix; a few lumps are okay.
4. Heat a non-stick skillet or griddle over medium heat and lightly coat with cooking spray or a small drizzle of olive oil.

5. Pour 1/4 cup of batter for each pancake onto the skillet. Cook for 2-3 minutes on each side or until pancakes are golden brown and cooked through.

6. Serve the pancakes warm, topped with Greek yogurt and drizzled with maple syrup.

Nutritional Information:

- Calories: Approximately 280 per serving
- Protein: 9 grams
- Fat: 3 grams (with minimal added fat for cooking)
- Carbohydrates: 53 grams
- Fiber: 6 grams
- Sugar: 20 grams (includes natural sugars from the bananas and added maple syrup)

Serving Size:

- Makes about 4 servings (2 pancakes per serving)

Cooking Time:

- Preparation time: 10 minutes
- Cook time: 6 minutes per batch of pancakes

Avocado Toast with Poached Eggs

Ingredients:

- 1 ripe avocado
- 2 eggs
- 2 slices of whole-grain bread
- 1 teaspoon of vinegar (for poaching eggs)
- Salt and pepper to taste
- Optional toppings: crushed red pepper, fresh herbs (such as cilantro or parsley), and a squeeze of lemon

Instructions:

1. Fill a medium saucepan with water, add vinegar, and bring to a gentle simmer.
2. Crack each egg into a small bowl. Gently slide the eggs one at a time into the simmering water. Cook for 3 to 4 minutes until the egg whites are set but yolks remain runny. Remove with a slotted spoon and set aside on a warm plate.
3. While eggs are poaching, toast the bread slices to your preferred crispness.
4. Halve the avocado and remove the pit. Scoop the avocado flesh into a bowl and mash with a fork. Season with salt, pepper, and a squeeze of lemon juice if desired.
5. Spread the mashed avocado evenly on each slice of toast.
6. Top each slice with a poached egg. Season with additional salt and pepper, and add any other desired toppings.

Nutritional Information:

- Calories: 290 per serving
- Total Fat: 20g
- Saturated Fat: 4g
- Cholesterol: 164mg
- Sodium: 400mg
- Carbohydrates: 20g
- Dietary Fiber: 7g
- Sugars: 3g
- Protein: 12g

Serving Size:

- 1 assembled avocado toast with one poached egg

Cooking Time:

- Preparation time: 10 minutes
- Cooking time: 5 minutes

Smoothie Bowl with Chia Seeds and Kiwi

Ingredients:

- 1 cup frozen mixed berries (blueberries, strawberries, raspberries)
- 1 ripe banana
- 1/2 cup unsweetened almond milk
- 1 tablespoon chia seeds
- 1 kiwi, peeled and sliced
- 1/4 cup sliced almonds
- 1 tablespoon honey (optional)

Instructions:

1. In a blender, combine the frozen berries, banana, and almond milk. Blend until smooth.
2. Pour the mixture into a bowl and stir in the chia seeds, letting sit for a few minutes to thicken.
3. Top the smoothie bowl with sliced kiwi, almonds, and a drizzle of honey if desired.

Nutritional Information:

- Calories: 285
- Sodium: 55 mg
- Fiber: 7 g
- Protein: 6 g

- Sugars: 20 g (natural sugars from fruits)

Serving Size:

This recipe serves one, making it a perfect single-serving breakfast that's easy to prepare and enjoy.

Cooking Time:

Preparation time is about 10 minutes, with no cooking required, making it a swift, no-fuss option for a nutritious start to the day.

Whole Wheat Blueberry Waffles

Ingredients:

- 1 cup whole wheat flour
- 1 tablespoon sugar
- 2 teaspoons baking powder
- 1/4 teaspoon salt
- 1 egg
- 1 cup non-fat milk
- 2 tablespoons vegetable oil
- 1/2 teaspoon vanilla extract
- 3/4 cup fresh blueberries

Instructions:

1. In a large mixing bowl, whisk together the whole wheat flour, sugar, baking powder, and salt.
2. In another bowl, beat the egg and then mix in the milk, vegetable oil, and vanilla extract.
3. Pour the wet ingredients into the dry ingredients and stir until just combined. Fold in the blueberries gently to avoid crushing them.
4. Heat a waffle iron and lightly grease it with cooking spray. Pour the batter onto the hot waffle iron, spreading it to the edges. Close the lid and cook according to the manufacturer's instructions until the waffle is golden and crisp.

5. Serve hot with a dollop of yogurt or a drizzle of honey if desired.

Nutritional Information (per serving):

- Calories: 210
- Fat: 8g
- Sodium: 200mg
- Carbohydrates: 30g
- Fiber: 4g
- Sugar: 8g
- Protein: 6g

Serving Size:

- Makes 4 waffles; serving size is 1 waffle.

Cooking Time:

- Prep time: 10 minutes
- Cook time: 5 minutes per waffle

Cottage Cheese with Pineapple and Chia

Ingredients:

- 1 cup low-fat cottage cheese
- 1/2 cup chopped fresh pineapple
- 1 tablespoon chia seeds
- Optional: a drizzle of honey or a sprinkle of cinnamon for added flavor

Instructions:

1. In a bowl, place the cottage cheese.
2. Top the cottage cheese with the chopped pineapple.
3. Sprinkle the chia seeds evenly over the pineapple.
4. If desired, add a light drizzle of honey or a dash of cinnamon for extra flavor.
5. Gently mix all the ingredients until well combined.
6. Serve immediately or chill in the refrigerator for 20 minutes to allow the chia seeds to swell slightly and the flavors to meld.

Nutritional Information:

Each serving of this dish provides approximately:
- Calories: 230
- Protein: 20 grams
- Fat: 8 grams (with minimal saturated fat)

- Carbohydrates: 20 grams
- Fiber: 4 grams
- Sodium: 500 mg

Serving Size:

This recipe makes 1 serving, making it easy to scale up if additional servings are needed.

Cooking Time:

Preparation time is about 5 minutes, with an optional chilling time of 20 minutes if a cooler breakfast is preferred.

Breakfast Quinoa with Apples and Cinnamon

Ingredients:

- 1 cup quinoa, rinsed
- 2 cups water
- 2 apples, peeled and diced
- 1/2 teaspoon ground cinnamon
- 1 tablespoon honey or maple syrup
- 1/4 cup chopped nuts (such as almonds or walnuts, optional)
- 1/4 cup low-fat milk or almond milk

Instructions:

1. In a small saucepan, combine quinoa and water. Bring to a boil over high heat.
2. Reduce heat to low, cover, and simmer until the quinoa is cooked and the water is absorbed, about 15 minutes.
3. Stir in the diced apples, cinnamon, and honey or maple syrup. Cook for another 5 minutes, or until the apples are soft.
4. Remove from heat and let sit, covered, for 5 minutes.
5. Fluff the quinoa with a fork and stir in the chopped nuts and milk.

Nutritional Information:

Each serving provides a balanced mix of carbohydrates, protein, and a modest amount of healthy fats. Specifically, it contains approximately:
- Calories: 250
- Protein: 6 grams
- Fat: 5 grams (with nuts, varies with type and amount of nuts used)
- Carbohydrates: 45 grams
- Fiber: 5 grams
- Sodium: 30 mg

Serving Size:

The recipe serves four, making it perfect for family breakfasts or preparing at the start of the week for a quick, reheatable meal option on busy mornings.

Cooking Time:

The total preparation and cooking time is about 25 minutes, making it an ideal choice for those seeking a nutritious, yet time-efficient, breakfast option.

Veggie Omelette with Mushrooms and Tomatoes

Ingredients:

- 2 eggs
- 1/4 cup low-fat milk
- 1/2 cup sliced mushrooms
- 1/2 cup chopped tomatoes
- 1/4 cup diced onions
- 1/4 teaspoon salt (optional)
- 1/4 teaspoon black pepper
- 1 teaspoon olive oil
- 1 tablespoon chopped fresh basil or parsley (for garnish)

Instructions:

1. In a medium bowl, whisk together the eggs, milk, salt (if using), and black pepper until well combined.

2. Heat the olive oil in a non-stick skillet over medium heat. Add onions and mushrooms, sautéing until the onions are translucent and mushrooms are golden, about 5 minutes.

3. Add the tomatoes and cook for another 2 minutes until the tomatoes are just soft.

4. Pour the egg mixture over the sautéed vegetables. Cook for about 4 minutes, or until the edges start to lift from the pan. Use a spatula to gently lift the edges and allow the uncooked egg to flow underneath.

5. Once the omelette is mostly set but slightly runny on top, fold it in half and allow it to cook for another minute.

6. Serve hot, garnished with fresh basil or parsley.

Nutritional Information:

- Calories: 210
- Total Fat: 12g (Saturated Fat: 3g)
- Cholesterol: 370mg
- Sodium: 230mg (if salt is added)
- Total Carbohydrates: 8g (Dietary Fiber: 2g, Sugars: 4g)
- Protein: 17g

Serving Size:

- This recipe serves 1, making it a perfect single-serving meal that's quick and easy to prepare.

Cooking Time:

- Total preparation and cooking time is approximately 20 minutes.

Chapter: 2 Lunch Recipes

Quinoa Salad with Chickpeas and Feta

For the Quinoa Salad with Chickpeas and Feta, you will need the following ingredients:

- 1 cup quinoa, rinsed
- 2 cups water
- 1 can (15 ounces) chickpeas, drained and rinsed
- 1 cucumber, diced
- 1 bell pepper, red or yellow, diced
- 1/2 red onion, finely chopped
- 1/2 cup crumbled feta cheese
- 1/4 cup chopped fresh parsley
- 3 tablespoons olive oil
- 2 tablespoons lemon juice
- 1 garlic clove, minced
- Salt and pepper to taste (keeping the salt minimal for DASH compliance)

Instructions for preparing this salad are straightforward:

1. In a medium saucepan, combine quinoa and water. Bring to a boil, then cover and reduce heat to simmer for about 15 minutes, or until water is absorbed and quinoa is tender.

2. Allow quinoa to cool to room temperature, then fluff with a fork.

3. In a large bowl, combine the cooked quinoa, chickpeas, cucumber, bell pepper, onion, and feta cheese.

4. In a small bowl, whisk together olive oil, lemon juice, minced garlic, salt, and pepper.

5. Pour the dressing over the salad and toss to combine. Stir in the chopped parsley.

6. Refrigerate the salad for at least 30 minutes to allow flavors to meld together before serving.

Nutritional Information for this dish (per serving):

- Calories: 265
- Total Fat: 10 g
- Saturated Fat: 3 g
- Cholesterol: 8 mg
- Sodium: 200 mg
- Total Carbohydrates: 34 g
- Dietary Fiber: 7 g
- Sugars: 5 g
- Protein: 10 g

The **Serving Size** for the Quinoa Salad with Chickpeas and Feta is approximately 1 cup, and this recipe typically makes about 6 servings.

The total **Cooking Time** includes about 15 minutes of cooking the quinoa and an additional 30 minutes of chilling time, making it a great option for meal prep or a quick, nutritious lunch option that can be enjoyed throughout the week.

Grilled Vegetable and Hummus Wraps

Ingredients:

- 1 zucchini, sliced lengthwise into thin strips
- 1 yellow bell pepper, deseeded and sliced into strips
- 1 red onion, sliced into rings
- 2 tablespoons olive oil
- Salt and pepper to taste
- 4 whole wheat tortillas
- 1 cup hummus
- 1/2 cup crumbled feta cheese
- 1/4 cup fresh basil leaves, chopped

Instructions:

1. Preheat the grill to medium-high heat. In a large bowl, toss the zucchini, bell pepper, and onion with olive oil, salt, and pepper until the vegetables are evenly coated.

2. Place the vegetables on the grill and cook for about 3-4 minutes on each side, or until they have nice grill marks and are tender. Remove from the grill and set aside to cool slightly.

3. Spread each tortilla evenly with hummus. Arrange the grilled vegetables evenly across the tortillas, and sprinkle with feta cheese and fresh basil.

4. Carefully roll up the tortillas tightly to enclose the fillings. You can serve them whole or cut in half, depending on preference.

5. Optionally, the wraps can be placed back on the grill for 1-2 minutes on each side to warm through and slightly crisp the tortilla.

Nutritional Information (per serving):

- Calories: 320
- Protein: 12g
- Fat: 17g
- Carbohydrates: 34g
- Fiber: 6g
- Sodium: 520mg

Serving Size:

- Makes 4 servings.

Cooking Time:

- Prep time: 10 minutes
- Cook time: 8 minutes

Turkey and Avocado Club Sandwich

Ingredients:

- 2 slices of whole-grain bread
- 4 ounces of thinly sliced turkey breast
- 1 ripe avocado, sliced
- 2 leaves of romaine lettuce
- 2 slices of tomato
- 1 tablespoon of low-fat mayonnaise
- 1 teaspoon of mustard
- Freshly ground black pepper, to taste

Instructions:

1. Toast the whole-grain bread slices lightly until they are just golden and crisp.
2. Spread the low-fat mayonnaise and mustard evenly over one side of each slice of bread.
3. On one slice of bread, layer the sliced turkey, followed by the tomato slices, romaine lettuce, and avocado.
4. Sprinkle the avocado with a pinch of black pepper to enhance its flavor.
5. Carefully place the second slice of bread on top, mayonnaise side down, to complete the sandwich.
6. Cut the sandwich diagonally into two triangles and serve immediately for the best taste and texture.

Nutritional Information:

- Calories: 370
- Total Fat: 15g
- Saturated Fat: 2g
- Cholesterol: 55mg
- Sodium: 420mg
- Carbohydrates: 32g
- Fiber: 8g
- Sugar: 5g
- Protein: 25g

Serving Size: 1 sandwich

Cooking Time: Approximately 10 minutes

Mixed Bean Soup with Barley

Ingredients:

- 1 cup of dried mixed beans (like kidney, black, and navy), soaked overnight and drained
- 1/2 cup pearled barley
- 1 large onion, diced
- 2 carrots, peeled and diced
- 2 celery stalks, diced
- 3 cloves of garlic, minced
- 1 teaspoon dried thyme
- 1 bay leaf
- 6 cups low-sodium vegetable broth
- 2 cups water
- Salt and freshly ground black pepper, to taste
- 2 tablespoons chopped fresh parsley

Instructions:

1. In a large pot, heat a splash of water or vegetable broth over medium heat. Add onions, carrots, and celery, and cook until they are softened, about 5 minutes.
2. Add the garlic, thyme, and bay leaf, and cook for another minute until fragrant.
3. Stir in the soaked and drained mixed beans and pearled barley.
4. Pour in the vegetable broth and water. Bring the mixture to a boil.

5. Reduce the heat to low and simmer, covered, for about 1 hour or until the beans and barley are tender.

6. Season with salt and pepper to taste. Remove the bay leaf before serving.

7. Garnish with fresh parsley.

Nutritional Information:

Each serving of this soup offers a balanced nutritional profile that supports cardiovascular health:

- Calories: Approximately 200 per serving
- Protein: 9 grams
- Fat: 1 gram
- Carbohydrates: 40 grams
- Fiber: 9 grams
- Sodium: Low sodium content, depending on the broth used

Serving Size:

This recipe serves 6 people. It's perfect for preparing a week's worth of lunches in advance, as the flavors continue to develop and improve while stored in the refrigerator.

Cooking Time:

The total preparation and cooking time for the Mixed Bean Soup with Barley is approximately 1 hour and 15 minutes. This includes the initial sautéing of vegetables, followed by about an hour of simmering to ensure that the beans and barley are fully cooked and the flavors are well blended.

Spinach and Strawberry Salad with Walnuts

The ingredients for the Spinach and Strawberry Salad with Walnuts are simple and readily available:

- 4 cups fresh spinach, washed and dried
- 1 cup fresh strawberries, sliced
- 1/2 cup walnuts, roughly chopped
- 1/4 cup crumbled feta cheese (optional)
- 2 tablespoons balsamic vinegar
- 1 tablespoon olive oil
- 1 teaspoon honey
- 1/4 teaspoon salt
- 1/4 teaspoon freshly ground black pepper

Instructions

To prepare the salad, start by whisking together balsamic vinegar, olive oil, honey, salt, and pepper in a large bowl to create the dressing. Add the spinach to the bowl and toss it gently to coat the leaves with the dressing. This ensures each bite is infused with flavor. Next, add the sliced strawberries and chopped walnuts to the spinach, and toss the ingredients lightly to combine. If you're using feta cheese, sprinkle it over the top of the salad before serving for a creamy textural contrast.

Nutritionally, this salad is a powerhouse. Each serving contains approximately:

- Calories: 210
- Fat: 15g
- Carbohydrates: 16g
- Fiber: 4g
- Protein: 5g
- Sodium: 170mg

Cooking time: 15 minutes

Tuna Salad Stuffed Tomatoes

Ingredients:

- 4 large ripe tomatoes
- 1 can (12 oz) tuna in water, drained
- 1/2 cup diced celery
- 1/4 cup finely chopped red onion
- 2 tablespoons chopped fresh parsley
- 1/4 cup low-fat Greek yogurt
- 1 tablespoon Dijon mustard
- 1 tablespoon lemon juice
- Salt and pepper to taste (keeping in mind the DASH diet's low sodium guidelines)

Instructions:

1. Cut the tops off the tomatoes and carefully scoop out the insides, leaving the walls intact. Invert the tomatoes on a paper towel to drain.

2. In a mixing bowl, combine the drained tuna, celery, red onion, and parsley. In a separate small bowl, whisk together Greek yogurt, Dijon mustard, and lemon juice to make a dressing.

3. Pour the dressing over the tuna mixture and stir until well combined. Season with a little salt and pepper, according to taste.

4. Spoon the tuna salad into the hollowed-out tomatoes. Chill in the refrigerator for at least 30 minutes before serving to allow flavors to meld.

Nutritional Information:

- Calories: 150 per serving
- Total Fat: 2g
- Saturated Fat: 0.5g
- Cholesterol: 30mg
- Sodium: 200mg
- Total Carbohydrates: 13g
- Dietary Fiber: 2g
- Sugars: 4g
- Protein: 20g

Serving Size:

- This recipe serves 4, with one stuffed tomato per serving.

Cooking Time:

- Preparation time: 15 minutes
- Chill time: 30 minutes

Chicken Caesar Salad with Whole Grain Croutons

Ingredients:

- 2 boneless, skinless chicken breasts
- 1 teaspoon olive oil
- Salt (minimal) and pepper to taste
- 4 cups of chopped Romaine lettuce
- 1 cup of cherry tomatoes, halved
- 1/2 cup of grated Parmesan cheese
- 1 cup whole grain bread, cut into cubes
- 2 cloves garlic, minced
- 1/4 cup low-fat Caesar dressing

Instructions:

1. Preheat the oven to 375°F (190°C).

2. Toss the bread cubes with olive oil and half of the minced garlic. Spread them on a baking sheet and bake for 10-15 minutes until crispy and golden. Set aside to cool.

3. While the croutons are baking, heat a grill pan over medium heat. Rub the chicken breasts with olive oil, salt, and pepper. Grill the chicken for 5-7 minutes on each side or until fully cooked and the juices run clear. Let the chicken rest for a few minutes before slicing it thinly.

4. In a large salad bowl, combine the chopped Romaine lettuce, cherry tomatoes, and sliced grilled chicken.

5. Add the whole grain croutons and Parmesan cheese to the salad.

6. Drizzle the low-fat Caesar dressing over the salad and toss to combine everything evenly.

7. Serve immediately for the best texture of the croutons and freshness of the salad.

Nutritional Information:

- Calories: 350 per serving
- Total Fat: 12g
- Saturated Fat: 3g
- Cholesterol: 75mg
- Sodium: 320mg
- Total Carbohydrates: 25g
- Dietary Fiber: 4g
- Sugars: 5g
- Protein: 35g

Serving Size:

- This recipe serves 2.

Cooking Time:

- Preparation time: 20 minutes
- Cooking time: 20 minutes
- Total time: 40 minutes

Mediterranean Veggie Pita Sandwich

Ingredients:

- 1 whole wheat pita bread
- 1/4 cup hummus
- 1/4 cucumber, thinly sliced
- 1 small tomato, thinly sliced
- 1/4 bell pepper, julienned
- 2 tablespoons red onion, thinly sliced
- 1/4 cup mixed greens (spinach, arugula, etc.)
- 2 tablespoons feta cheese, crumbled
- 1 tablespoon olives, sliced
- 1 teaspoon olive oil
- 1/2 teaspoon dried oregano
- Salt and pepper to taste (keep salt minimal to align with DASH guidelines)

Instructions:

1. Cut the pita bread in half to make two pockets and gently open each half to create space for the fillings.
2. Spread hummus evenly inside each pita half.
3. Layer cucumber, tomato, bell pepper, red onion, and mixed greens inside each pita.
4. Sprinkle feta cheese and olives on top of the vegetables.
5. Drizzle olive oil over the filling and season with oregano, salt, and pepper.

6. Serve immediately or wrap in foil to maintain freshness for a packed lunch.

Nutritional Information:

- Calories: 300
- Total Fat: 9g
- Saturated Fat: 2g
- Cholesterol: 8mg
- Sodium: 320mg
- Total Carbohydrates: 45g
- Dietary Fiber: 6g
- Sugars: 5g
- Protein: 12g

Serving Size:

- Serves 1 (2 pita halves per serving)

Cooking Time:

- Preparation Time: 10 minutes
- Total Time: 10 minutes

Butternut Squash and Apple Soup

Ingredients:

- 1 tablespoon olive oil
- 1 medium onion, chopped
- 2 cloves garlic, minced
- 1 butternut squash (about 2 pounds), peeled, seeded, and cubed
- 2 large apples, peeled, cored, and chopped (preferably a tart variety like Granny Smith)
- 4 cups low-sodium vegetable broth
- 1 teaspoon ground cinnamon
- ½ teaspoon ground nutmeg
- Salt and pepper to taste
- Fresh chives, chopped (for garnish)

Instructions:

1. Heat the olive oil in a large pot over medium heat. Add the onion and garlic, sautéing until the onions become translucent.
2. Add the cubed butternut squash and chopped apples to the pot, stirring to combine.
3. Pour in the vegetable broth, ensuring that the squash and apples are fully submerged. Bring the mixture to a boil.
4. Reduce heat to low and simmer for about 25-30 minutes, or until the squash and apples are very tender.

5. Use an immersion blender to puree the soup directly in the pot until smooth. Alternatively, carefully transfer the soup in batches to a blender to puree.

6. Stir in the cinnamon, nutmeg, salt, and pepper. Adjust the seasonings to taste.

7. Serve hot, garnished with chopped chives.

Nutritional Information (per serving):

- Calories: 160
- Fat: 2.5g
- Saturated Fat: 0.4g
- Cholesterol: 0mg
- Sodium: 120mg
- Carbohydrates: 35g
- Fiber: 6g
- Sugar: 12g
- Protein: 2g

Serving Size: This recipe serves 4, making it ideal for family meals or preparing ahead for multiple days.

Cooking Time: Preparation takes about 15 minutes, with a cooking time of approximately 30 minutes. Total time from start to finish is around 45 minutes, making it a feasible option for a healthy, home-cooked lunch even on a busy day.

Roasted Beet and Citrus Salad

Ingredients:

- 4 medium beets, peeled and diced
- 2 oranges, peeled and segments segmented
- 1 grapefruit, peeled and segments segmented
- 2 tablespoons of olive oil
- Salt and pepper to taste
- 2 teaspoons of honey (optional)
- 1/4 cup chopped walnuts
- 1/2 red onion, thinly sliced
- Fresh mint leaves for garnish

Instructions:

1. Preheat your oven to 400°F (200°C).
2. Toss the diced beets in one tablespoon of olive oil and season with salt and pepper. Spread them on a baking sheet and roast for about 30-40 minutes until tender and slightly caramelized.
3. In a large bowl, combine the roasted beets, orange and grapefruit segments, red onion, and chopped walnuts.
4. Whisk together the remaining olive oil, a pinch of salt, pepper, and honey if using, to create a dressing.
5. Drizzle the dressing over the salad and toss gently to coat all the ingredients.
6. Garnish with fresh mint leaves before serving.

Nutritional Information:

- Calories: 200
- Total Fat: 10g
- Saturated Fat: 1.5g
- Cholesterol: 0mg
- Sodium: 150mg
- Total Carbohydrates: 27g
- Dietary Fiber: 6g
- Sugars: 18g
- Protein: 4g

Serving Size:

This recipe serves 4, making it an ideal dish for a family lunch or to be portioned out for individual meals throughout the week.

Cooking Time:

The total preparation and cooking time is approximately 50 minutes, with most of this being the beet roasting time, which is mostly hands-off.

Chapter: 3 Dinner Recipes

Baked Salmon with Dill and Lemon

Ingredients:

- 4 salmon fillets (6 ounces each)
- 2 tablespoons olive oil
- 1 tablespoon fresh dill, chopped
- 1 lemon, thinly sliced
- Salt and pepper to taste

Instructions:

1. Preheat your oven to 400°F (200°C).
2. Line a baking sheet with parchment paper and place the salmon fillets skin-side down.
3. Brush each fillet with olive oil and season with salt and pepper.
4. Sprinkle chopped dill evenly over the fillets and top each with a few lemon slices.
5. Bake in the preheated oven for 12-15 minutes or until the salmon flakes easily with a fork.

Nutritional Information per serving:

- Calories: 295
- Fat: 17g
- Saturated Fat: 2.5g

- Cholesterol: 77mg
- Sodium: 75mg
- Carbohydrates: 1g
- Fiber: 0.2g
- Protein: 34g

Serving Size: This recipe serves 4, with each serving consisting of one 6-ounce fillet.

Cooking Time: The total time required, including preparation and cooking, is approximately 20 minutes.

Grilled Chicken with Quinoa and Broccoli

Ingredients:

- 4 boneless, skinless chicken breasts
- 1 cup quinoa
- 2 cups broccoli florets
- 2 tablespoons olive oil
- 1 teaspoon minced garlic
- 1 lemon, juiced and zested
- 1 teaspoon dried thyme
- Salt and pepper to taste (keeping in mind the low sodium goal of the DASH diet)

Instructions:

1. Rinse the quinoa under cold water until the water runs clear. In a medium saucepan, bring 2 cups of water to a boil. Add the quinoa, cover, and reduce the heat to low. Simmer for 15 minutes or until the water is absorbed. Remove from heat and let sit, covered, for 5 minutes. Fluff with a fork.

2. While the quinoa is cooking, preheat the grill to medium-high heat. Rub the chicken breasts with 1 tablespoon of olive oil, lemon zest, thyme, salt, and pepper.

3. Place the chicken on the grill and cook for 6-7 minutes on each side, or until the internal temperature reaches 165°F (75°C).

4. In a separate pan, heat the remaining olive oil over medium heat. Add garlic and sauté for about 30 seconds, or until fragrant. Add the broccoli florets and sauté for about 5 minutes, or until they are tender and vibrant green. Season with lemon juice and a pinch of salt and pepper.

5. Serve the grilled chicken sliced on top of a bed of quinoa and side of sautéed broccoli.

Nutritional Information (per serving):

- Calories: 350
- Fat: 10g
- Carbohydrates: 30g
- Fiber: 5g
- Protein: 35g
- Sodium: 150mg

Serving Size: This recipe serves 4 people.

Cooking Time: The total cooking time is approximately 30 minutes, making it an ideal quick dinner option for busy evenings.

Vegetable Stir-Fry with Tofu and Brown Rice

Ingredients:

- 1 block of firm tofu, drained and cubed
- 2 cups brown rice, cooked
- 1 tablespoon olive oil
- 2 cloves garlic, minced
- 1 red bell pepper, sliced
- 1 cup broccoli florets
- 1 cup snap peas
- 1 carrot, julienned
- 2 tablespoons low-sodium soy sauce
- 1 tablespoon sesame oil
- 1 teaspoon fresh ginger, grated
- 1 tablespoon cornstarch mixed with 2 tablespoons water
- Fresh cilantro, for garnish
- Sesame seeds, for garnish

Instructions:

1. Prepare the brown rice according to package instructions.
2. In a large skillet or wok, heat the olive oil over medium-high heat. Add the tofu and sauté until golden brown on all sides,

approximately 5-7 minutes. Remove the tofu from the skillet and set aside.

3. In the same skillet, add a bit more oil if needed, and sauté garlic, red bell pepper, broccoli, snap peas, and carrot until they begin to soften, about 5 minutes.

4. Return the tofu to the skillet. Stir in the low-sodium soy sauce, sesame oil, and grated ginger. Cook for another 2-3 minutes, letting the flavors meld.

5. Stir the cornstarch and water mixture into the skillet. Cook for another 2 minutes, or until the sauce has thickened slightly.

6. Serve the stir-fry over the cooked brown rice, garnished with fresh cilantro and sesame seeds.

Nutritional Information:

- Calories: 330
- Fat: 12g
- Saturated Fat: 2g
- Carbohydrates: 44g
- Fiber: 5g
- Protein: 18g
- Sodium: 300mg

Serving Size:

- This recipe serves 4 people.

Cooking Time:

- Preparation time: 15 minutes
- Cooking time: 20 minutes

Beef Stew with Root Vegetables

Ingredients:

- 1 lb lean beef chuck, cut into cubes
- 2 tablespoons olive oil
- 1 medium onion, chopped
- 2 cloves garlic, minced
- 2 carrots, peeled and diced
- 2 parsnips, peeled and diced
- 1 sweet potato, peeled and cubed
- 1 turnip, peeled and cubed
- 4 cups low-sodium beef broth
- 1 bay leaf
- 1 teaspoon dried thyme
- Salt (optional) and pepper to taste
- 2 tablespoons fresh parsley, chopped (for garnish)

Instructions:

1. Heat the olive oil in a large pot over medium-high heat. Add the beef cubes and sear until all sides are browned, about 5-7 minutes. Remove the beef and set aside.

2. In the same pot, add the onion and garlic, cooking until they are translucent, about 3 minutes.

3. Return the beef to the pot along with carrots, parsnips, sweet potato, turnip, beef broth, bay leaf, and thyme. Bring to a boil.

4. Once boiling, reduce heat to a simmer and cover the pot. Let it cook for about 1.5 hours or until the beef and vegetables are tender.

5. Remove the bay leaf, season with salt (if using) and pepper to taste. Garnish with fresh parsley before serving.

Nutritional Information (per serving):

- Calories: 310
- Protein: 26 g
- Fat: 15 g
- Carbohydrates: 22 g
- Fiber: 4 g
- Sodium: 180 mg

Serving Size:

- Makes about 4 servings.

Cooking Time:

- Prep time: 20 minutes
- Cook time: Approximately 1.5 hours

Pasta Primavera with a Light Tomato Sauce

Ingredients:

- 8 oz whole grain spaghetti or fettuccine
- 2 tablespoons olive oil
- 1 small onion, finely chopped
- 2 garlic cloves, minced
- 1 zucchini, sliced into half-moons
- 1 yellow bell pepper, sliced into thin strips
- 1 cup cherry tomatoes, halved
- 1 cup fresh spinach leaves
- 1/2 cup low-sodium vegetable broth
- 1 cup canned crushed tomatoes
- 1 teaspoon dried basil
- 1 teaspoon dried oregano
- Salt and pepper, to taste
- Fresh basil, for garnish

Instructions:

1. Cook pasta according to package instructions until al dente; drain and set aside.
2. In a large skillet, heat olive oil over medium heat. Add onion and garlic, sautéing until the onion is translucent.
3. Add zucchini and bell pepper to the skillet, sautéing for about 5 minutes until just tender.

4. Stir in cherry tomatoes and spinach, cooking until the spinach is wilted.

5. Pour in vegetable broth and crushed tomatoes, bringing the mixture to a simmer.

6. Season with dried basil, oregano, salt, and pepper. Let simmer for an additional 5 minutes to allow flavors to meld.

7. Toss the cooked pasta with the sauce, ensuring it is evenly coated.

8. Serve hot, garnished with fresh basil.

Nutritional Information (per serving):

- Calories: 320
- Fat: 7g
- Saturated Fat: 1g
- Cholesterol: 0mg
- Sodium: 150mg
- Carbohydrates: 55g
- Fiber: 10g
- Sugar: 8g
- Protein: 10g

Serving Size:

- This recipe serves 4.

Cooking Time:

- Total preparation and cooking time is approximately 30 minutes.

Pork Tenderloin with Roasted Sweet Potatoes

Ingredients:

- 1 lb pork tenderloin
- 2 large sweet potatoes, peeled and cubed
- 1 tbsp olive oil
- 1 tsp smoked paprika
- 1 tsp garlic powder
- 1/2 tsp ground black pepper
- 1/4 tsp salt
- Fresh thyme, a few sprigs

Instructions:

1. Preheat your oven to 375°F (190°C).
2. In a small bowl, combine the smoked paprika, garlic powder, salt, and black pepper.
3. Rub the pork tenderloin with half of the olive oil and then coat evenly with the spice mixture.
4. In a separate bowl, toss the cubed sweet potatoes with the remaining olive oil and a pinch of salt and pepper.
5. Place the pork tenderloin in the center of a baking sheet and arrange the sweet potatoes around it. Scatter a few sprigs of thyme over the pork and potatoes.

6. Roast in the preheated oven for about 25-30 minutes, or until the pork reaches an internal temperature of 145°F (63°C) and the sweet potatoes are tender.

7. Remove from oven, let the pork rest for 5 minutes, and then slice.

Nutritional Information per Serving:

- Calories: 295
- Total Fat: 10g
- Saturated Fat: 2g
- Cholesterol: 75mg
- Sodium: 210mg
- Total Carbohydrates: 23g
- Dietary Fiber: 3g
- Sugars: 5g
- Protein: 28g

Serving Size:

- This recipe serves 4, with each serving consisting of approximately 4 oz of pork and a half-cup of roasted sweet potatoes.

Cooking Time:

- Total preparation and cooking time is approximately 40 minutes, which includes the resting time for the pork to ensure it is juicy and tender.

Seafood Paella with Brown Rice

Ingredients:

- 1 tablespoon olive oil
- 1 onion, finely chopped
- 2 cloves garlic, minced
- 1 red bell pepper, diced
- 1 cup brown rice
- 1/4 teaspoon saffron threads
- 1/2 teaspoon smoked paprika
- 2 tomatoes, diced
- 4 cups low-sodium vegetable broth
- 1 cup frozen peas
- 1 pound mixed seafood (shrimp, scallops, and mussels), cleaned
- 1/4 cup chopped fresh parsley
- 1 lemon, cut into wedges

Instructions:

1. Heat the olive oil in a large skillet or paella pan over medium heat. Add the onion and garlic, and sauté until the onion is translucent.
2. Add the red bell pepper and cook for another 3 minutes.
3. Stir in the brown rice, saffron threads, and smoked paprika until well combined with the aromatics.
4. Mix in the diced tomatoes and cook for 2 minutes before pouring in the vegetable broth. Bring the mixture to a boil.

5. Reduce the heat to low, cover, and simmer for about 30 minutes, or until the rice is almost tender.

6. Add the frozen peas and mixed seafood, spreading the seafood evenly throughout the pan. Cover and cook for an additional 10 minutes, or until the seafood is thoroughly cooked and the rice is tender.

7. Remove from heat and let the paella sit, covered, for 5 minutes to absorb any remaining liquid.

8. Garnish with chopped parsley and serve with lemon wedges on the side.

Nutritional Information (per serving):

- Calories: 350
- Fat: 6g
- Sodium: 200mg
- Carbohydrates: 44g
- Fiber: 5g
- Protein: 25g

Serving Size:

- This recipe serves 4 people.

Cooking Time:

- Total preparation and cooking time is approximately 55 minutes.

Eggplant Parmesan Light

Ingredients:

- 2 large eggplants, sliced into 1/2 inch rounds
- 2 cups marinara sauce, low sodium
- 1 cup shredded mozzarella cheese, part-skim
- 1/4 cup grated Parmesan cheese, reduced fat
- 1/2 cup whole wheat breadcrumbs
- 2 eggs, beaten
- 1/4 cup fresh basil, chopped
- 2 cloves garlic, minced
- Olive oil spray
- Salt and pepper to taste

Instructions:

1. Preheat the oven to 375 degrees Fahrenheit. Lightly spray a baking sheet with olive oil spray.
2. Dip eggplant slices in beaten eggs, then coat with breadcrumbs seasoned with minced garlic, salt, and pepper. Arrange slices on the baking sheet and spray the tops lightly with olive oil.
3. Bake the eggplant for 25 minutes, turning once until both sides are golden and crisp.
4. In a baking dish, spread a thin layer of marinara sauce. Layer half of the baked eggplant slices over the sauce. Sprinkle half of the mozzarella and Parmesan cheeses over the eggplant. Repeat with another layer of sauce, eggplant, and cheeses.

5. Cover with foil and bake in the oven for 20 minutes. Remove the foil and bake for another 10 minutes or until the cheese is bubbly and golden.

6. Garnish with fresh basil before serving.

Nutritional Information:

Per serving, the Eggplant Parmesan Light provides approximately:

- Calories: 290

- Fat: 9g (Saturated Fat: 4g)

- Sodium: 320mg

- Carbohydrates: 38g (Fiber: 11g, Sugars: 14g)

- Protein: 19g

Serving Size:

The recipe serves 6, with each serving consisting of 2 to 3 slices of eggplant, covered in sauce and cheese, making it a filling and nutritious dinner option.

Cooking Time:

The total cooking time is approximately 55 minutes, with 25 minutes for baking the eggplant and 30 minutes for assembling and baking the layered dish.

Turkey Chili with Beans

Ingredients:

- 1 lb ground turkey (lean)
- 1 large onion, chopped
- 2 cloves garlic, minced
- 2 tablespoons chili powder
- 1 teaspoon ground cumin
- 1 can (28 ounces) no-salt-added diced tomatoes
- 1 can (15 ounces) kidney beans, rinsed and drained
- 1 can (15 ounces) black beans, rinsed and drained
- 1 green bell pepper, chopped
- 1 red bell pepper, chopped
- 2 cups low-sodium chicken broth
- Salt and pepper to taste
- Optional toppings: chopped fresh cilantro, sliced green onions, or a dollop of low-fat sour cream

Instructions:

1. In a large pot, cook the ground turkey over medium heat until browned, stirring to crumble. Drain any excess fat.
2. Add the chopped onion and garlic to the pot and cook until the onions are translucent.
3. Stir in chili powder and cumin, cooking for another minute to release the flavors.

4. Add the diced tomatoes, kidney beans, black beans, green and red bell peppers, and chicken broth. Season with salt and pepper to taste.

5. Bring the mixture to a boil, then reduce heat and simmer uncovered for about 30 minutes, stirring occasionally.

6. Serve hot, garnished with optional toppings if desired.

Nutritional Information:

Each serving of Turkey Chili with Beans provides a balanced nutritional profile ideal for a heart-healthy diet:

- Calories: 250
- Protein: 20g
- Fat: 5g (Saturated Fat: 1g)
- Carbohydrates: 30g (Dietary Fiber: 8g; Sugars: 5g)
- Sodium: 300mg

Serving Size:

This recipe serves 6 people, making it perfect for family dinners or for having leftovers for the next day.

Cooking Time:

Preparation time for this recipe is approximately 10 minutes, with a cooking time of 40 minutes. This brings the total time to about 50 minutes from start to finish.

Lentil and Spinach Curry

Ingredients:

- 1 tablespoon olive oil
- 1 large onion, finely chopped
- 2 cloves garlic, minced
- 1 tablespoon freshly grated ginger
- 1 tablespoon curry powder
- 1 teaspoon ground cumin
- 1/2 teaspoon ground turmeric
- 1/4 teaspoon cayenne pepper (optional, adjust to taste)
- 1 cup dried brown lentils, rinsed
- 4 cups low-sodium vegetable broth
- 3 cups fresh spinach leaves, roughly chopped
- 1 tablespoon fresh lemon juice
- Salt to taste (optional, monitor for a low-sodium diet)

Instructions:

1. Heat the olive oil in a large saucepan over medium heat. Add the onion and cook until translucent, about 5 minutes.
2. Add the garlic and ginger, cooking for another minute until fragrant.
3. Stir in the curry powder, cumin, turmeric, and cayenne pepper, and cook for another minute to release the flavors.

4. Add the rinsed lentils and vegetable broth. Bring to a boil, then reduce the heat to low, cover, and simmer for about 25 minutes, or until the lentils are tender.

5. Stir in the chopped spinach and continue to cook until the spinach wilts, about 3 minutes.

6. Remove from heat and stir in the lemon juice. Adjust seasoning with salt if needed.

7. Serve warm.

Nutritional Information (per serving):

- Calories: 210
- Total Fat: 3g
- Saturated Fat: 0.5g
- Cholesterol: 0mg
- Sodium: 70mg
- Total Carbohydrates: 32g
- Dietary Fiber: 15g
- Sugars: 3g
- Protein: 13g

Serving Size:

This recipe yields four servings, making it perfect for a family meal or for preparing ahead for multiple meals.

Cooking Time:

Total preparation and cooking time is approximately 40 minutes.

Chapter: 4 Snacks and Sides

Healthy Snack Options

1. Cucumber Hummus Bites

Ingredients:

- 1 large cucumber, sliced into rounds
- 1 cup hummus
- Cherry tomatoes, halved
- Fresh parsley, chopped

Instructions:

- Arrange cucumber slices on a platter.
- Spoon a dollop of hummus on each cucumber slice.
- Top each with a half cherry tomato and sprinkle with parsley.

Nutritional Information:

- Calories: 35 per bite
- Fat: 1.5g
- Sodium: 80mg
- Carbohydrates: 4g
- Protein: 2g

Serving Size: 1 bite

2. Greek Yogurt and Berry Parfait

Ingredients:
 - 1 cup plain Greek yogurt
 - ½ cup mixed berries (blueberries, raspberries, strawberries)
 - 2 tbsp honey
 - ¼ cup granola

Instructions:
 - In a glass, layer half the Greek yogurt, followed by half the mixed berries and a drizzle of honey.
 - Repeat the layering with the remaining yogurt, berries, and honey.
 - Top with granola before serving.

Nutritional Information:
 - Calories: 210
 - Fat: 2g
 - Sodium: 55mg
 - Carbohydrates: 36g
 - Protein: 15g

Serving Size: 1 parfait

Cooking Time: No cooking required

3. Avocado Toast with Radishes

Ingredients:

- 2 slices whole grain bread
- 1 ripe avocado
- 4 radishes, thinly sliced
- Lemon juice, salt, and pepper to taste

Instructions:

- Toast the bread slices to your preferred doneness.
- Mash the avocado and spread evenly on each slice of toast.
- Top with radish slices, then sprinkle with lemon juice, salt, and pepper.

Nutritional Information:

- Calories: 250 per slice
- Fat: 15g
- Sodium: 200mg
- Carbohydrates: 27g
- Protein: 6g

Serving Size: 1 slice

Cooking Time: 5 minutes

4. Spiced Nuts

Ingredients:

- 1 cup raw mixed nuts (almonds, walnuts, pecans)
- 1 tsp olive oil
- ½ tsp chili powder
- ½ tsp cumin
- ¼ tsp salt

Instructions:

- Preheat oven to 350°F (175°C).
- In a bowl, mix nuts with olive oil, chili powder, cumin, and salt.
- Spread nuts on a baking sheet and bake for 10-12 minutes, stirring once.

Nutritional Information:

- Calories: 170 per ¼ cup
- Fat: 15g
- Sodium: 80mg
- Carbohydrates: 6g
- Protein: 5g

Serving Size: ¼ cup

Cooking Time: 12 minutes

Sides to Complement Your Meals

1. Crispy Kale Chips

Ingredients:
- 1 bunch kale, washed and dried
- 1 tablespoon olive oil
- 1/4 teaspoon salt

Instructions:
- Preheat oven to 350°F (175°C).
- Remove the ribs from the kale and cut into 1 1/2-inch pieces.
- Toss kale with olive oil and salt, then spread on a baking sheet.
- Bake for 10-15 minutes or until crispy.

Nutritional Information:
- Calories: 58
- Fat: 2.5g
- Sodium: 150mg
- Carbohydrates: 7.3g
- Fiber: 1.3g
- Protein: 2.2g

Serving Size: 4 servings

Cooking Time: 15 minutes

2. Quinoa and Black Bean Salad

Ingredients:

- 1 cup quinoa
- 2 cups water
- 1 can (15 ounces) black beans, drained and rinsed
- 1 red bell pepper, chopped
- 1/4 cup fresh cilantro, chopped
- 1 lime, juiced
- 2 tablespoons olive oil
- 1/2 teaspoon ground cumin
- Salt and pepper to taste

Instructions:

- In a saucepan bring water to a boil. Add quinoa and a pinch of salt. Reduce to a simmer, cover, and cook until all water is absorbed, about 15 minutes.
- Let quinoa cool, then mix with black beans, bell pepper, cilantro, lime juice, olive oil, cumin, salt, and pepper.

Nutritional Information:

- Calories: 222
- Fat: 7g
- Sodium: 13mg
- Carbohydrates: 33g
- Fiber: 8g

- Protein: 9g

Serving Size: 6 servings

Cooking Time: 20 minutes

3. Garlic and Herb Roasted Carrots

Ingredients:
- 6 large carrots, peeled and sliced into batons
- 2 tablespoons olive oil
- 3 cloves garlic, minced
- 2 tablespoons chopped fresh parsley
- 1 teaspoon chopped fresh thyme
- Salt and pepper to taste

Instructions:
- Preheat oven to 400°F (200°C).
- Toss carrots with olive oil, garlic, parsley, thyme, salt, and pepper.
- Spread on a baking sheet and roast for 25-30 minutes until tender and lightly caramelized.

Nutritional Information:
- Calories: 120
- Fat: 7g

- Sodium: 86mg
  - Carbohydrates: 14g
  - Fiber: 4g
  - Protein: 1g

Serving Size: 4 servings

Cooking Time: 30 minutes

Chapter: 5 Desserts

Sweet Treats That Fit the DASH Diet

1. Banana Berry Sorbet

Ingredients:

- 2 ripe bananas
- 1 cup frozen mixed berries (strawberries, blueberries, raspberries)
- 1 tablespoon honey (optional)
- 2 tablespoons water

Instructions:

1. Peel and slice bananas.
2. In a blender, combine bananas, frozen berries, honey (if using), and water.
3. Blend until smooth.
4. Freeze the mixture for at least 3-4 hours until firm.
5. Serve chilled.

Nutritional Information (per serving):

- Calories: 110
- Fat: 0.3g
- Sodium: 3mg

- Carbohydrates: 28g

- Fiber: 3g

- Protein: 1.2g

Serving Size: 1/2 cup

Cooking Time: 4 hours (including freezing time)

2. Almond Joy Oatmeal Cookies

Ingredients:
- 1 cup rolled oats
- 1/2 cup whole wheat flour
- 1/3 cup unsweetened shredded coconut
- 1/2 teaspoon baking soda
- 1/4 teaspoon salt
- 1/4 cup unsalted almonds, chopped
- 1/4 cup dark chocolate chips
- 1/4 cup unsweetened applesauce
- 1/4 cup honey
- 1 egg

Instructions:
1. Preheat oven to 350°F (175°C).
2. In a large bowl, mix oats, flour, coconut, baking soda, and salt.
3. Stir in almonds and chocolate chips.

4. In another bowl, combine applesauce, honey, and egg.

5. Mix wet ingredients into dry ingredients until well combined.

6. Drop tablespoon-sized portions onto a baking sheet.

7. Bake for 10-12 minutes or until cookies are golden brown.

Nutritional Information (per serving):
- Calories: 150
- Fat: 7g
- Sodium: 80mg
- Carbohydrates: 21g
- Fiber: 2g
- Protein: 3g

Serving Size: 1 cookie

Cooking Time: 12 minutes

3. Cinnamon Apple Crisp

Ingredients:
- 4 medium apples, peeled, cored, and sliced
- 1 teaspoon ground cinnamon
- 2 tablespoons brown sugar
- 1/2 cup rolled oats
- 1/4 cup whole wheat flour
- 1/4 cup unsalted butter, melted

- 1/4 cup chopped walnuts

Instructions:

1. Preheat oven to 375°F (190°C).

2. In a large bowl, toss apple slices with cinnamon and brown sugar.

3. Spread apples in a baking dish.

4. In the same bowl, mix oats, flour, butter, and walnuts until crumbly.

5. Sprinkle the oat mixture over the apples.

6. Bake for 30 minutes or until the topping is golden and apples are tender.

Nutritional Information (per serving):

- Calories: 220
- Fat: 10g
- Sodium: 5mg
- Carbohydrates: 34g
- Fiber: 5g
- Protein: 3g

Serving Size: 1/2 cup

Cooking Time: 30 minutes

Chapter: 6 Drinks and Beverages

Refreshing Drinks for Hydration and Health

1. Cucumber Mint Water

Ingredients:
- 1 large cucumber, thinly sliced
- 10 fresh mint leaves
- 2 quarts of water

Instructions:
- Combine cucumber and mint in a large pitcher.
- Fill the pitcher with water and stir gently.
- Refrigerate for at least 4 hours or overnight to enhance the flavors.

Nutritional Information (per serving):
- Calories:
- Fat: 0g
- Carbohydrates: 0g
- Protein: 0g

Serving Size: 1 cup

Cooking Time: 0 minutes (4+ hours refrigerating)

2. Lemon Ginger Tea

Ingredients:
- 1 inch ginger root, peeled and thinly sliced
- 2 tablespoons honey
- Juice of 1 lemon
- 4 cups water

Instructions:
- In a saucepan, bring water and ginger to a boil.
- Simmer for 15 minutes.
- Remove from heat and add lemon juice and honey, stirring until honey dissolves.
- Strain into cups.

Nutritional Information (per serving):
- Calories: 50
- Fat: 0g
- Carbohydrates: 13g
- Protein: 0g

Serving Size: 1 cup

Cooking Time: 20 minutes

3. Berry and Flaxseed Smoothie

Ingredients:
- 1 cup mixed berries (blueberries, strawberries, raspberries)
- 1 tablespoon ground flaxseed
- 1 cup low-fat yogurt
- ½ cup unsweetened almond milk

Instructions:
- Place all ingredients in a blender.
- Blend on high until smooth.

Nutritional Information (per serving):
- **Calories: 150**
- Fat: 4g
- Carbohydrates: 24g
- Protein: 6g

Serving Size: 1 cup

Cooking Time: 5 minutes

4. Herbal Citrus Iced Tea

Ingredients:

- 4 cups water
- 2 herbal tea bags (e.g., chamomile or peppermint)
- Juice of 1 orange
- Juice of 1 lemon
- 1 tablespoon honey

Instructions:

- Bring water to a boil and steep tea bags for about 5 minutes.
- Remove tea bags and add citrus juices and honey.
- Stir well and chill.
- Serve over ice.

Nutritional Information (per serving):

- Calories: 25
- Fat: 0g
- Carbohydrates: 6g
- Protein: 0g

Serving Size: 1 cup

Cooking Time: 10 minutes (plus chilling time)

Conclusion

Embarking on the journey presented in the "DASH Diet Cookbook For Beginners 2024" is more than just adopting a new set of eating habits; it's about embracing a lifestyle change that prioritizes your health and well-being. This cookbook serves as a comprehensive guide that not only introduces you to nutritious recipes but also educates you on the reasons behind each dietary choice and how they benefit your overall health. It provides the tools and knowledge necessary to navigate a path toward reduced blood pressure and improved heart health.

Throughout this cookbook, the focus has been on easy-to-follow recipes enriched with whole grains, lean proteins, and plenty of fruits and vegetables, all aligned with the DASH diet's principles. By reducing sodium intake and increasing nutrients like potassium and magnesium, these meals help manage and prevent hypertension. The inclusion of various recipes ensures that everyone, regardless of their culinary skill level or time constraints, can find dishes that fit their lifestyle.

The additional sections on meal planning and ingredient substitutions further empower you to take control of your diet by making informed decisions that suit your specific needs and preferences. This adaptability is crucial in maintaining a sustainable diet that doesn't feel restrictive but rather enriching and enjoyable.

Moreover, the cookbook's guidance on how to effectively use kitchen tools and understand ingredient labels prepares you to make healthier choices beyond the recipes provided. These skills are valuable in any cooking scenario and encourage a more mindful approach to eating and health.

As you continue to use this cookbook, you'll likely find that the benefits extend beyond just dietary changes. Many find improvements in their energy levels, general wellness, and even mental health. The simple act of taking time to prepare wholesome, delicious meals can be a meditative practice that reduces stress and enhances your quality of life.

In conclusion, the "DASH Diet Cookbook For Beginners 2024" is not merely a collection of recipes; it's a gateway to a healthier lifestyle. The habits you develop from this cookbook are designed to last a lifetime, offering a foundation of knowledge that supports continuous improvement and a vibrant, healthful future. By embracing the lessons and recipes it provides, you're not just cooking; you're committing to a healthier, happier you.